The 15 Best Arm Toning Exercises for Women [Illustrated]

30 Days to Firmer, Toned & Sexy Arms [Fitness Model Physique Series]

Rachel Howe

NORDICSTANDARD PUBLISHING

Atlanta, Georgia USA
ISBN 978-1-48396-815-5

9 781483 968155 >

D1597422

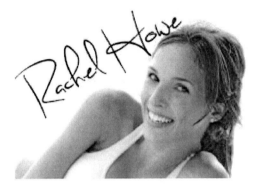

Copyright © 2012 Rachel Howe

What Our Readers Are Saying

"I have always wanted great looking arms, but could never get a workout plan that would make a difference. The combination that Rachel Howe lays out in her book finally did the trick. My arms now look great, but also the top half of my body feels wonderful."

★★★★★**Joyce Waldron (Salt Lake City, UT)**

"There is no way how I can explain what this book did for me. I never had the patience for my arms before and felt that age and gravity were just going to take its toll. Finally with a proper diet and these workouts, my arms look better than they did when I was 20."

★★★★★**Frances Lancaster (Franklin, TN)**

"Howe has put together a really good guide. I added this workout to my own, and I have seen a real improvement around my upper arms and shoulders. I also experience much less back pain."

★★★★★Betty D Langdon (Atlanta, GA)

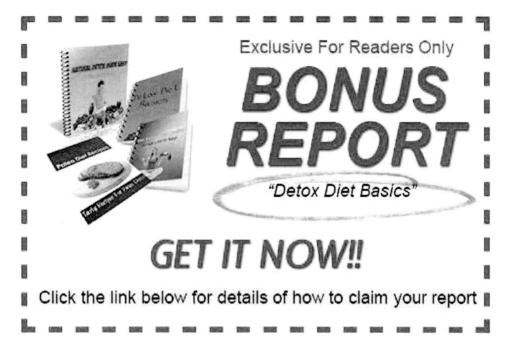

Exclusive Bonus Download: Detox Diet Basics

Our internal organs, the colon, liver and intestines, help our bodies eliminate toxic and harmful matter from our bloodstreams and tissues. Often, our systems become overloaded with waste.

The very air we breathe, and all of its pollutants, build up in our bodies.

Today's over processed foods and environmental pollutants can easily overwhelm our delicate systems and cause toxic matter to build up in our bodies.

Go to the end of this book for the download link for this Bonus

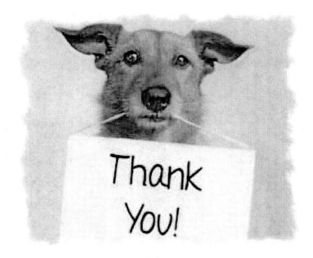

Thank you for downloading my book. Please REVIEW this book on Amazon. I need your feedback to make the next version better. Thank you so much!

Books by Rachel Howe

THE 15 BEST BREAST LIFTING EXERCISES FOR WOMEN [ILLUSTRATED]

THE BEST BUTT EXERCISES FOR WOMEN

THE 12 BEST THIGH TONING EXERCISES FOR WOMEN

THE TOP 10 BEST CALF TONING EXERCISES FOR WOMEN [ILLUSTRATED]

THE 15 BEST ARM TONING EXERCISES FOR WOMEN [ILLUSTRATED]

www.amazon.com/author/rachel-howe

Why You Should Read This Book

THE 15 BEST ARM TONING EXERCISES FOR WOMEN is the ideal book for any woman that has always desired firm, toned arms that accentuate any dress or sleeveless top. When your arms are in shape, you feel younger about yourself and to some degree braver. Thanks to Rachel Howe you will have the perfect arm workout ready to use on a daily basis.

Never again worry about having to keep your arms covered up out of embarrassed. Rid yourself of that feeling with the 15 exercises put together in this book especially for you. You will love the results the next time you put on that sleeveless top. When you add this workout to your own routine, you will have the strong and toned arms that will look great in any outfit.

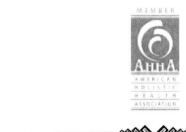

TABLE OF CONTENTS

Disclaimer

While all attempts have been made to provide effective, verifiable information in this Book, neither the Author nor Publisher assumes any responsibility for errors, inaccuracies, or omissions. Any slights of people or organizations are unintentional.

This Book is not a source of medical information, and it should not be regarded as such. This publication is designed to provide accurate and authoritative information in regard to the subject matter covered. It is sold with the understanding that the publisher is not engaged in rendering a medical service. As with any medical advice, the reader is strongly encouraged to seek professional medical advice before taking action.

The 15 Best Arm Toning Exercises

Toned shoulders and arms not only help to keep a woman feeling fit, they also help to keep her feeling and looking younger. There can be no doubt that saggy arms or sloping shoulders add years to a woman's appearance and while it may be true that muscle tone naturally changes with advancing years, it's absolutely not true that nothing can be done about it! Muscle tone can be improved at any age or stage in life and all it takes is a healthy diet and a program of regular exercise to achieve the definition in your arm muscles that allows you to wear even the most summery of sleeveless or strapless outfits with confidence.

To tone up your arms, you need to target the main muscle groups of triceps, biceps, and shoulders. The triceps form the back of your upper arm and they are exercised through pushing movements, the biceps form the front of your upper arm and they are exercised through pulling movements, and your shoulders are exercised each time you raise your arm away from your body. The following exercises are all designed to target specific muscle groups or a combination of muscles so pick and choose from the list to add variety to your arm workout.

1. Triceps Extensions

As its name suggests, this exercise targets the triceps muscles on the back of your upper arms. The exercise can be performed using a dumbbell or any suitable hand-held weight and it can be done one arm at a time or both arms together as shown in the illustrations below.

- Stand with your feet placed hip-width apart and then move one foot slightly forward to achieve a solid base for maintaining your balance.

- Hold the weight overhead with straight arms.

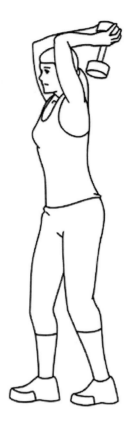

- Position your elbows at shoulder-width apart and keep good posture throughout your body with your head, neck, and spine in line.

- Slowly bend your elbows, maintaining control of the weight, until you reach a 90 degree angle in your elbow joint, or as far as you can lower the weight without allowing your upper arms to move from the upright position.

- Take care not to hit your head with the weight!

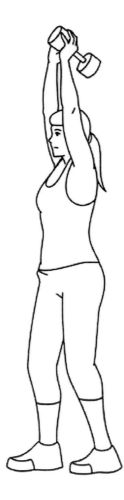

- Slowly raise the weight back to the overhead starting position.

- Repeat the movements to complete one set of 12 to 15 repetitions before allowing your arms a short rest. Complete a second set of 12 to 15 repetitions.

- Breathe normally throughout the exercise.

2. Triceps Kickbacks

Triceps kickbacks also target the triceps muscles and are performed one arm at a time. Single arm exercises provide the added benefit of addressing any muscle imbalances in your body as both arms must work individually without any support from other muscles. This means that weak triceps in one arm cannot be "carried" by stronger triceps in the other arm, creating greater symmetry across your upper body.

- Position yourself with one knee and one hand on a bench as illustrated below.

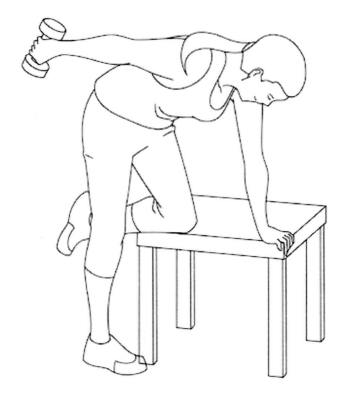

- Hold the dumbbell (or other hand-held weight) in the other hand and position your arm with a bent elbow and the back of your upper arm in line with the line of your back as shown. It's important to keep your head, neck, and spine in line, so it can be helpful to look down at the floor.

- Straighten your elbow to "kickback" the weight without allowing your upper arm to move from its starting position.

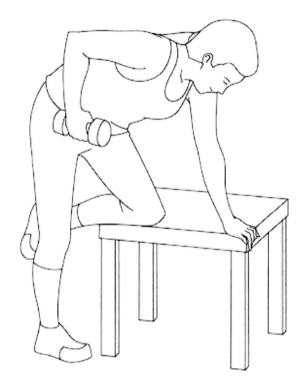

- Slowly return the weight to the starting position; repeat the kickback.

- Complete one set of 12 to 15 repetitions using your right arm then switch positions to complete one set of 12 to 15 repetitions using your left arm.

- Complete a second set of 12 to 15 repetitions with each arm.

- Breathe normally throughout the exercise.

3. Triceps Dips

An alternative exercise to target the triceps muscles is the triceps dip. Only bodyweight is used in this exercise but it's important to ensure the chair, bench, step, or any solid object you use is fixed in position.

- Sit on a bench or chair which is pushed against a wall or heavy enough not to move as you exercise.

- Position your hands on either side of your body and grip the bench or chair.

- Move your feet and body forward so that your bodyweight is being supported by your arms.

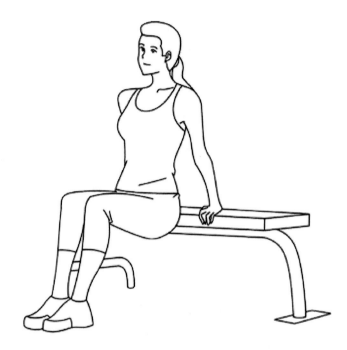

- Bend your elbows to allow your butt to move slowly toward the floor (but not so low that you sit down!)

- Straighten your elbows to lift your body back up to bench level (but again, don't sit down!) Keep a slight bend in your elbows at the end of the movement to avoid straining your joints.

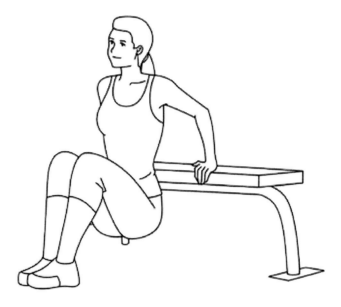

- Repeat the movements to complete one set of 12 to 15 repetitions before allowing yourself to sit down for a rest. Complete a second set of 12 to 15 repetitions.

- Breathe normally throughout the exercise.

- Experiment with different foot positions. The further away from the bench you place your feet, the greater the intensity of the exercise.

4. Push-Up Against a Wall

The standard push-up exercise targets the triceps muscle groups of your upper arm and also the pectoral muscles of your chest. In this version of the push-up, the intensity of the exercise is lowered to make the movements more manageable but the effectiveness of the workout on the targeted muscle groups remains the same. The additional benefit of any push-up exercise is the workout given to your core postural muscles.

- Stand facing a wall at around arms-length away with your feet placed hip-width apart.

- Lean in toward the wall and place your hands against it at shoulder-height and width apart.

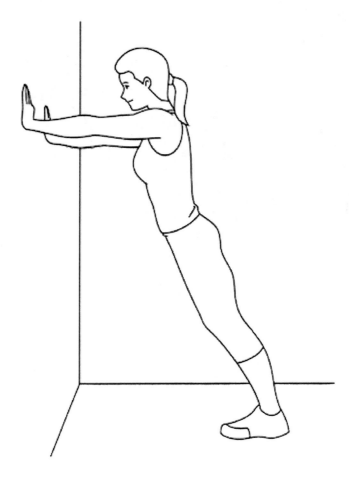

- Push back from the wall to straighten your arms. Keep a slight bend in your elbows at the end of the movement to prevent potential joint strain.

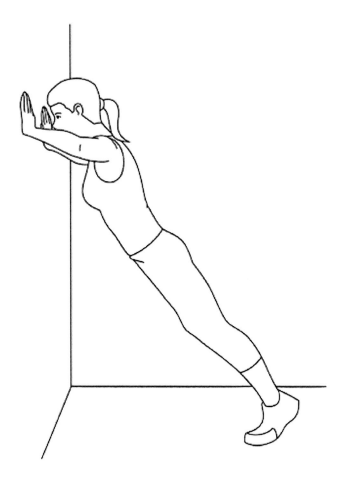

- Repeat the movements to complete one set of 12 to 15 repetitions before taking a short rest. Complete a second set of 12 to 15 repetitions.

- Maintain good posture and breathe normally throughout the exercise.

5. Incline Push-Up

This version of the push-up exercise is slightly more intense than the push-up against a wall exercise above and therefore it increases the workload on the working muscle groups of triceps and pectorals. The incline push-up provides a natural progression from the wall push-up when you're ready for a new challenge.

- Position yourself in the start position as illustrated. Any solid object of a suitable height can be used in place of a bench. A kitchen counter provides a useful alternative.

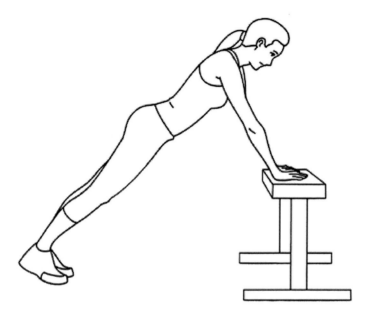

- Place your hands at shoulder-width or slightly wider apart.

- Maintain good posture throughout your body with head, neck, and spine in line.

- Bend your elbows to lower your chest toward the bench. Control the movement and breathe normally throughout.

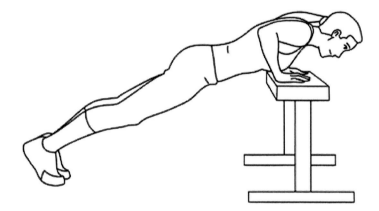

- Push back from the bench by straightening your arms. Keep a slight bend in your elbows at the end of the movement to avoid joint strain.

- Repeat the movements to complete one set of 12 to 15 repetitions before taking a short rest. Complete a second set of 12 to 15 repetitions.

6. Push-Up on Knees

This version of the push-up exercise provides further progression from the incline push-up exercise above.

- Position yourself on the floor on your hands and knecs as illustrated below.

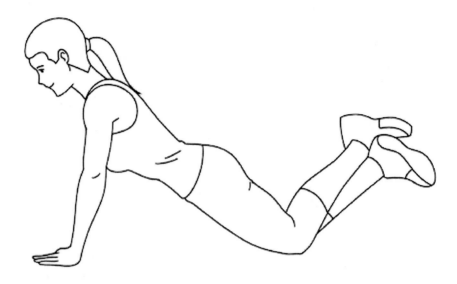

- Place your hands under your shoulders at around shoulder-width or slightly wider apart. Raise your feet from the floor by crossing your ankles.

- Slowly lower your chest toward the floor by bending your elbows. Maintain good posture throughout your body with your head, neck, and spine in line.

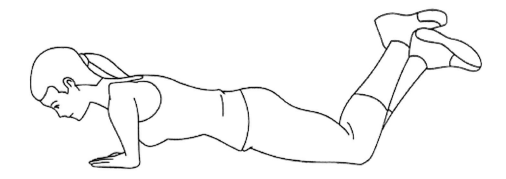

- Push up from the floor by straightening your arms. Keep a slight bend in your elbows at the end of the movement to avoid the potential for joint strain.

- Repeat the movements to complete one set of 12 to 15 repetitions before taking a short rest. Complete a second set of 12 to 15 repetitions.

- Breathe normally throughout the exercise.

7. Push-Up on Gym Ball

This decline version of the push-up exercise adds a further challenge for the working muscle groups. The workload of the triceps and pectorals is increased and the core muscles of your lower back along with your abdominals work harder to help you maintain your balance and posture.

- Roll across the top of a gym ball on your stomach to place your hands on the floor on the other side.

- Move your body forward on the ball so that the majority of your weight is taken by your arms. Experiment with starting positions to find the correct degree of challenge for you. The further from the ball you place your hands, the greater the intensity of the exercise.

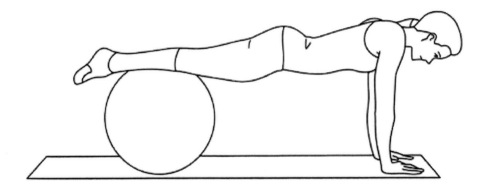

- Maintain good posture by keeping your head in line with your neck and your neck in line with your spine.

- Bend your elbows to lower your chest toward the floor.

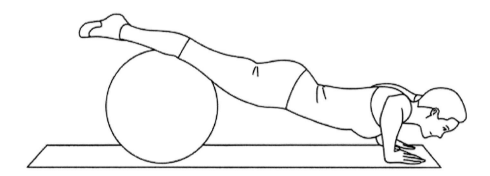

- Push back up by straightening your arms. Keep a slight bend in your elbows at the end of the movement to prevent joint strain.

- Repeat the movements to complete one set of 12 to 15 repetitions before taking a short rest. Complete a second set of 12 to 15 repetitions.

- Breathe normally throughout the exercise and go slowly to stay in control of all movements.

8. Shoulder Press

The shoulder press exercise targets the triceps muscle groups as well as the muscles of your shoulders. It can be performed with dumbbells or any other suitable hand-held weights, including an exercise band. It can be done from a seated position or a standing position as illustrated below.

- Stand with your feet placed hip-width apart.

- Raise the weights to shoulder height (but not resting on your shoulders) and position your hands so that your wrists and palms face inwards.

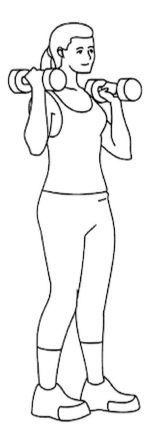

- Raise the weights overhead by straightening your arms, keeping them at shoulder-width apart. Keep a slight bend in your elbows at the end of the movement to minimize the stress placed on the joints.

- Maintain good posture in your body throughout, with your head, neck, and spine in line. Avoid any body swinging, tilting, or arching of your back as you lift the weights.

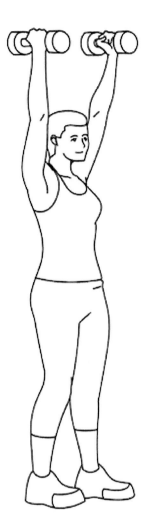

- Slowly lower the weights back to shoulder height; repeat the exercise.

- Aim to complete one set of 12 to 15 repetitions before taking a short rest. Complete a second set of 12 to 15 repetitions.

- Breathe normally throughout the exercise.

9. Lateral Raises

Lateral raises target the muscles of your shoulders and specifically the center portion of the muscle group. This exercise can be performed with dumbbells or any other suitable hand-held weights, including an exercise band, and it can also be done in a seated position as well as a standing position as illustrated below.

- Stand with your feet placed hip-width apart.

- Hold the weights in front of your body with wrists and palms facing toward each other.

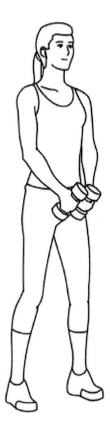

- Keeping your arms "straight," raise the weights out to the side of your body until they reach shoulder height. The aim is to allow your elbows to lead the way in the lift, not your wrists, and it's important to keep a slight bend in your "straight" arm position to avoid the potential for elbow joint strain.

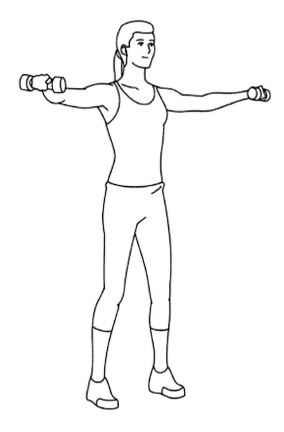

- Slowly return the weights to the starting position, controlling the movement at every stage.

- Repeat the movements to complete one set of 12 to 15 repetitions before taking a short rest. Complete a second set of 12 to 15 repetitions.

- Breathe normally throughout the exercise and maintain good posture. Avoid any body tilting or arching of your back as you raise the weights.

10. Front Raises

This exercise also targets the shoulder muscles but specifically the front portion of the muscle group. It can be performed with dumbbells, a barbell, or any other suitable hand-held weight, including an exercise band.

- Stand with your feet placed hip-width apart and place one foot slightly further forward to achieve a solid base for maintaining your balance.

- Hold the weights in front of your thighs with your wrists and palms facing toward your body.

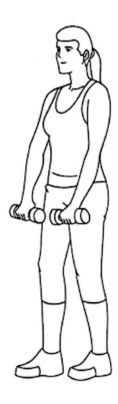

- Keep the weights at shoulder-width apart and raise them with a "straight" arm to shoulder height. It's important to keep a slight bend in your elbows to avoid the potential for joint strain when using weights.

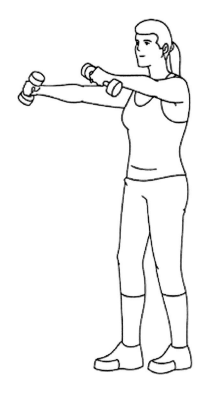

- Maintain good posture throughout the lift, avoiding any temptation to swing your body or arch your back to aid the lift.

- Slowly lower the weights back to the starting position, keeping control of the movement at every stage.

- Repeat the movements to complete one set of 12 to 15 repetitions before taking a short rest. Complete a second set of 12 to 15 repetitions.

- Breathe normally throughout the exercise.

11. Upright Row

The upright row is a pulling exercise so in addition to working the shoulders it also recruits the biceps muscles on the front of your upper arm. It can be performed with dumbbells, a barbell, or any suitable hand-held weights, including an exercise band.

- Stand with feet placed hip-width apart.

- Hold the weights in front of your body with wrists and palms facing towards your thighs. Allow the weights to touch ends (or your thumbs to touch if holding a barbell.)

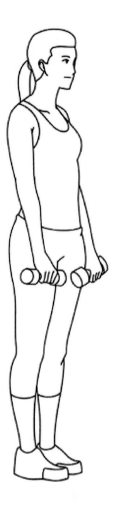

- Raise the weights straight up the line of your body to just under chin height, allowing your elbows to lead the way.

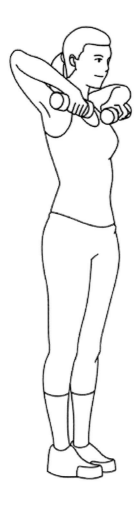

- Slowly return the weights to the starting position, staying in control of the movement at every stage.

- Maintain good posture throughout with your head, neck, and spine in line. It's important to avoid any body rocking or back arching in an effort to aid the lift.

- Repeat the movements to complete one set of 12 to 15 repetitions before taking a short rest. Complete a second set of 12 to 15 repetitions.

- Breathe normally throughout the exercise.

12. Bicep Curls

As its name suggests, this exercise targets the biceps muscles on the front of your upper arms. It can be performed in a seated position with dumbbells or in a standing position with dumbbells or a barbell. Stand with feet placed hip-width apart.

- Hold the weights in front of your thighs with your palms and wrists facing away from your body.

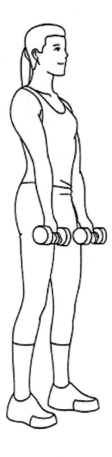

- Lift the weights towards your shoulders by bending your elbows. It's important to keep your elbows in place by your sides and to maintain your upper arm position. Only your lower arms should move.

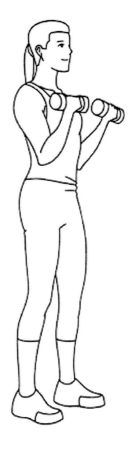

- Slowly return the weights to the starting position, staying in control of the movement at every stage.

- Repeat the movements to complete one set of 12 to 15 repetitions before taking a short rest. Complete a second set of 12 to 15 repetitions.

- Maintain good posture throughout the exercise. Your head, neck, and spine must remain in line and any temptation to swing your body to aid the lift avoided.

- Breathe normally, focusing on maintaining good posture by pulling your shoulders back if they have a natural tendency to round and pulling your tummy button toward your spine to create a strong core.

13. Alternate Arm Bicep Curls

One advantage of using dumbbells in the bicep curl is that the exercise can be performed with both arms together or one arm at a time, with an alternating arm movement allowing one arm to rest while the other arm works.

- Maintaining good posture, perform one complete bicep curl repetition with your right arm followed by one complete repetition with your left arm.

- Continue to alternate arms until each arm has completed 15 repetitions in total before taking a short rest.

- Repeat the exercise to complete a further 15 repetitions with each arm.

- Add variety by completing one bicep curl repetition with your right arm followed by one repetition with your left arm followed by a double arm bicep curl.

14. Seated Row

The seated row can be performed on gym equipment designed to target your biceps and the rhomboid muscles between your shoulder blades. The same exercise can also be performed at home using an exercise band.

- Position yourself on the floor as in the illustration below with the exercise band in place around the soles of your feet and held in both hands.

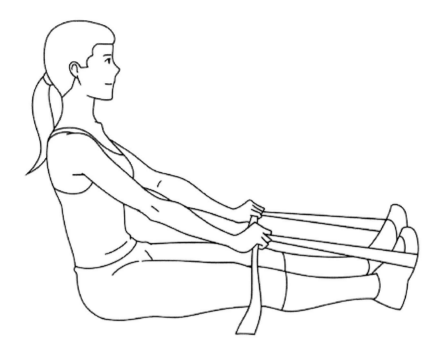

- Using a rowing action, bend your elbows to feel the resistance of the band. It's important that only your arms move and that your upper body remains still and upright.

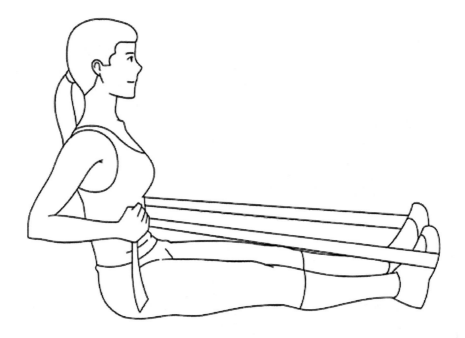

- Allow your arms to return slowly to the starting position, maintaining control of the movement at all stages.

- Repeat the movements to complete one set of 12 to 15 repetitions before taking a short rest. Complete a second set of 12 to 15 repetitions.

- Breathe normally throughout the exercise and avoid any upper body movements such as leaning back in an effort to assist the rowing action. Experiment with different exercise band lengths and tensions to find the correct level of challenge for you.

15. Upright Row, Front Raise, Shoulder Press Combo

Using dumbbells, combine the upright row, front raise, and shoulder press exercises to create an all-round arm toning workout. Alternate the movements by performing one complete upright row repetition followed by one complete front raise repetition followed by one complete shoulder press repetition until you have completed your chosen total number of repetitions. The upright row tones the center portion of your shoulders and your biceps, the front raise tones the front portion of your shoulders, and the shoulder press tones your triceps along with your shoulders.

It's important to remain in control of all movements and to make the change from one exercise to the next slowly and methodically to ensure that correct form is used each time. Controlled movements which target specific muscle groups are of far greater benefit than "cheating" movements such as body swinging which use momentum rather than muscle!

Exclusive Bonus Download: Detox Diet Basics

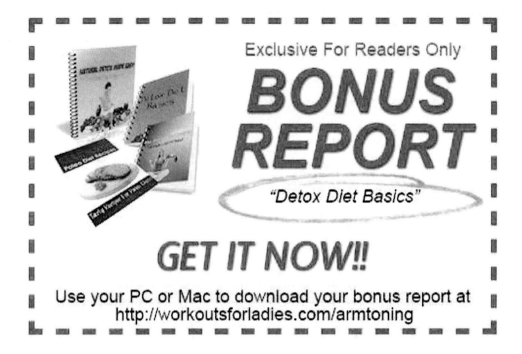

Download your bonus, please visit the download link above from your PC or MAC. To open PDF files, visit http://get.adobe.com/reader/ to download the reader if it's not already installed on your PC or Mac. To open ZIP files, you may need to download WinZip from http://www.winzip.com. This download is for PC or Mac ONLY and might not be downloadable to kindle.

Our internal organs, the colon, liver and intestines, help our bodies eliminate toxic and harmful matter from our bloodstreams and tissues. Often, our systems become overloaded with waste.

The very air we breathe, and all of its pollutants, build up in our bodies.

Today's over processed foods and environmental pollutants can easily overwhelm our delicate systems and cause toxic matter to build up in our bodies.

Visit the URL above to download this guide and start improving your body NOW

One Last Thing...

Thank you so much for reading my book. I hope you really liked it. As you probably know, many people look at the reviews on Amazon before they decide to purchase a book. If you liked the book, could you please take a minute to leave a review with your feedback? 60 seconds is all I'm asking for, and it would mean the world to me.

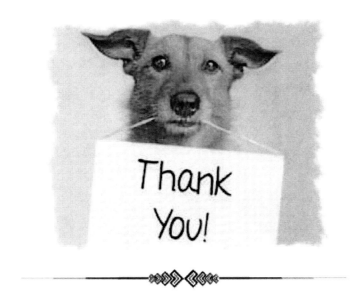

Books by Rachel Howe

THE 15 BEST BREAST LIFTING EXERCISES FOR WOMEN [ILLUSTRATED]

THE BEST BUTT EXERCISES FOR WOMEN

THE 12 BEST THIGH TONING EXERCISES FOR WOMEN

THE TOP 10 BEST CALF TONING EXERCISES FOR WOMEN [ILLUSTRATED]

THE 15 BEST ARM TONING EXERCISES FOR WOMEN [ILLUSTRATED]

www.amazon.com/author/rachel-howe

About Rachel Howe

Rachel Howe is a personal trainer, author and competitive triathlete from California. She holds a master of science degree in exercise and sport science in addition to a number of fitness industry certifications and accreditations.

She has one daughter and a loving husband. She is an healthy eating enthusiast and her spare time she can often be found either cooking, jogginh, hiking or cycling with the family.

Rachel Howe

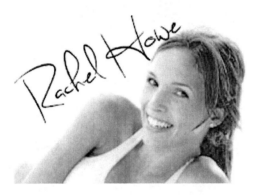

Images and Cover by Nordic Standard Publishing

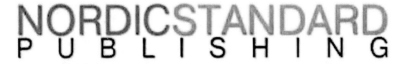

Atlanta, Georgia USA

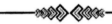

CPSIA information can be obtained
at www.ICGtesting.com
Printed in the USA
LVOW09s1311220917
549726LV00004B/159/P

Laughter Therapy

Discover How To Use Laughter And Humor For Healing, Stress Relief, Improved Health, Increased Emotional Wellbeing, And A More Joyful and Happy Life

By Ace McCloud
Copyright © 2013

Disclaimer

The information provided in this book is designed to provide helpful information on the subjects discussed. This book is not meant to be used, nor should it be used, to diagnose or treat any medical condition. For diagnosis or treatment of any medical problem, consult your own physician. The publisher and author are not responsible for any specific health or allergy needs that may require medical supervision and are not liable for any damages or negative consequences from any treatment, action, application or preparation, to any person reading or following the information in this book. Any references included are provided for informational purposes only. Readers should be aware that any websites or links listed in this book may change.

Table of Contents

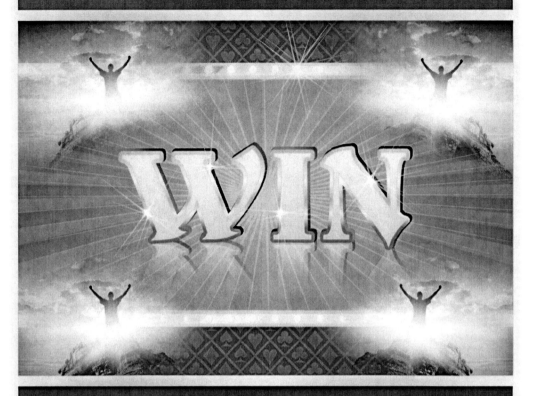

DEDICATED TO THOSE WHO ARE PLAYING THE GAME OF LIFE TO

WIN

KEEP ON PUSHING AND NEVER GIVE UP!

Ace McCloud

Be sure to check out my website for all my Books and Audio books.

www.AcesEbooks.com

Introduction

I want to thank you and congratulate you for buying the book, "Laughter and Humor Therapy: Learn How To Use Laughter And Humor For Healing, Stress Relief, Improved Health, Increased Emotional Wellbeing, And A More Joyful and Happy Life."

This book contains proven steps and strategies on how to successfully incorporate laughter into your everyday life for a happier and healthier you. You will also discover the facts about the physical and psychological benefits of laughter, as well as the various ways to incorporate laughter into your everyday life. Also included are proven exercises and therapies for overcoming depressed moods and for creating a sense of enjoyment and mirth that may be missing from your life. Be sure that you are utilizing one of the greatest stress relievers and natural therapies of all time in your every day life!

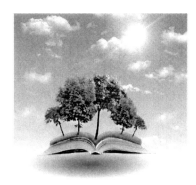

Chapter 1: Laugh out Loud- Here's Why!

Call it chucking, chortling, giggling, or hee-hawing; we all know what laughter is. Some of the best moments all of us remember throughout our lives are the times when we've laughed to our heart's content. People go to great efforts to find enjoyment through laughter. To make other people laugh we write books, we watch comedic films and sitcoms, we go to comedy clubs, we research jokes to impress our friends and family, and much more. A good comedian can make millions of dollars just by making people laugh. We like to laugh because laughing feels good. But did you know that laughing has actual mental and physical benefits?

The benefits of laughter date back thousands of years. For instance, in ancient Greece, physicians were known to send their patients to the Hall of Comedians to relieve symptoms such as depression, pain, and broken hearts. Native Americans also knew the health benefits of humor, and they considered the clown the third most important person in their tribe. The clown would often accompany the witch doctor on important meetings with those who were suffering or in pain. In the 1300's, the surgeon Henri de Mondeville, would visit his patients in the recovery room and tell them jokes, considering his surgery incomplete unless he made his patients laugh. Much later, in the 20th century, clowns were sent to hospitals to visit children suffering from polio. There are many stories throughout history of the healing power of laughter.

Laughter is still in use for medical benefits today. In our modern age, when we are able to systematically collect and analyze data, we know for certain that laughter is good for us. Laughter has been shown to boost T-cells, which helps the body protect against sickness. Laughter is also good for the heart. Laughter increases blood flow to the heart, decreases inflammation, and reduces platelet aggregation. It also relieves stress by eliciting the release of endorphins.

Humans aren't the only species that laughs. Other primates, such as chimpanzees, have been shown to laugh. This shows that laughter has been in our genes for a very long time. Behavioral Evolutionists believe that laughter developed in the Savannah, to indicate when a danger had passed. It also serves as a social cue. People rarely laugh when they are by themselves, and almost everyone finds laughter contagious. This was soon realized by sitcom producers in the 1950's, when they started putting laugh tracks as a background in their episodes and using live audiences.

Laughter is a way of relieving tension and letting others know that things are okay. For instance, a stranger might give a polite laugh if you accidently close a door on them or a nervous interviewee may laugh a little in hopes that the interviewer might laugh back, expressing that the interview is going well.

Chapter 2: Laughter in Life

Have you noticed how often babies and children laugh? It may seem strange, but they have the innate ability of finding humor in many situations. The fact is, as people mature, they carry much more responsibilities and emotional baggage. By the time we reach adulthood, we laugh only about twenty times a day. Meanwhile, babies laugh about three hundred times a day!

You may also notice that babies and children never miss an opportunity to make fun of a situation. They feel free to make themselves look silly or even try to turn a lot of boring conversation into jokes. We should try walking in those tiny shoes and start actively trying to create moments of mirth and giggles. Here are some quick and easy ways to add humor into your life:

Be around people who make you laugh
Sigmund Freud would recommend to his depressed patients to surround themselves with people who made them laugh. If you hang around someone with a similar sense of humor, you'll be more likely to find many more things funny and laughter will come that much more easily. Also, laughter is contagious. Just being in the same room with people laughing in it can start you up.

Simulate social environments
Studies have shown people are much more likely to laugh when reading a book, watching television, and while playing video games, than in more isolated surroundings. This is because the TV or computer can simulate a social setting, making laughter much easier to come by.

Get in some kid time
Babysit your friend's child or spend more time with your little relatives. As stated earlier, children laugh much more than adults. Laughter is one of the most positive benefits of young children! Go ahead and have some laughs with them!

Make time to laugh
You read that right. You don't have to dedicate a whole night to laughing (although it does sound like a fun idea, doesn't it?). You can squeeze in the time throughout the day by *creating* humor. Try this, the next time you're in a serious board meeting, imagine something completely ridiculous happening like your boss farting, or a coworker quitting in an extravagant way. You could also try singing along to a funny song on the way to work, or buying a book filled with jokes. Many newspapers have a section solely devoted to humor and comics.

Expose Yourself to Humorous Media
This is simple enough. The next time you are choosing a movie pick a comedy over a drama. If you are picking a restaurant, pick a fun restaurant, like a place with a happy atmosphere and lots of games. Look for jokes on the internet or funny videos on YouTube. If you put in the effort, there are thousands of choices

we can make to increase our chances of finding humor and laughter in our everyday life.

Chapter 3: Laughter-The Alternative Way

Alternative and complementary medicine practices are gaining increased popularity and acceptance all around the world, and many people are now choosing them as legitimate options to improve their health and wellbeing. It turns out, that these therapies may help you to improve your mental health by encouraging you to look at the positive side of life and by encouraging you to actively look for joy and laughter. Let's have a quick look at some of the best alternative medicine therapies that could help you get into a better frame of mind so that you can laugh your worries away, or simply smash them into oblivion!

Chakra Healing
One of the most popular, yet controversial forms of alternative medicine, is chakra healing. It is an interesting philosophy of healing that deals with the 7 major 'chakras' of the body. Basically, the chakras are nothing but spinning wheels of energy located at 7 different points on the body, each of them dealing with a specific bodily function.

Ideally, in a state of complete health, an individual has all of his or her chakras spinning correctly. If there is imbalance in the body, like disease or injury, this is said to be clearly reflected in the chakras. While chakras are not really visible to the naked human eye, they can be visualized and 'felt' when experts look through their mind's eye.

Stress, depression, and other mental disorders are said to be easily handled using chakra therapy. Chakra therapy is a natural approach to treating various disorders. It is believed that the throat chakra has the most to do with mental disorders, since the throat is the home to the thyroid gland, which in fact, deals with your emotional stability.

While the chakras may not really be visible to everyone, getting the chakras in balance is not that hard to do. Start by sitting in a comfortable position and breathing in deeply through the nose. Let your breath out through your mouth. The simple act of breathing is a great stress buster, and it is also great for calming down frazzled nerves, making you less prone to anxiety, mood swings and depression.

Next, place the palm of your right hand on your throat, and the palm of the left hand directly on your belly button- and move your focus to the throat region, warding away any mental chatter you may have. Now, as you breathe deeply, imagine the throat region getting filled with golden light particles that contain amazing healing energies, moving in a circle around your throat, illuminating the area around you. Hold this mental image for as long as you can, preferably as long as you feel 'good' doing it.

Doing this exercise regularly has been thought to facilitate the removal of toxins, revitalize the thyroid gland, and improve the thyroid gland's overall function.

When this is done, it can have a positive impact on your mental well-being, and it is less likely that you will fall prey to anxiety, stress, and other disorders. In this more enlightened frame of mind, laughter and humor should come much easier to you.

Acupressure/Acupuncture
Acupuncture and acupressure have their roots dating back to the ancient times, and these practices, which fall under the tradition of Chinese medicine, are still being used today to help many people manage their various conditions.

Both of these practices work on the same principle- the life force energy (qi), which flows through the body, is responsible for the health or the disease of an individual. This energy, which flows through the various channels of the body, helps provide energy and helps to keep all of the bodies organs functioning properly.

On the other hand, it is said that clogging in the movement of these energies throughout the body can be potentially dangerous, and can help enable the occurrence of many diseases and health problems.

If you're looking to assess your mental problems, like insomnia, anxiety, stress, worry, and depression, without the use of anti-depressants and other drugs, these therapies work wonderfully for many different people.

By stimulating certain points on the body, the flow of energy through the body can be restored, the blockages can be removed, and you can experience an overall sense of well-being.

Patients suffering from various mental illnesses have reported feeling better after an acupuncture/acupressure session, and they tend to laugh (and enjoy their lives) more often.

Make sure you visit a qualified professional to seek acupuncture/acupressure services to get the best out of your session.

Yoga and Deep Breathing Exercises
Yoga and deep breathing exercises hold many benefits that we all know about. These benefits have been talked about in newspapers, magazines, books, tv shows, dvd's, and more. Yoga and deep breathing exercises are great for rejuvenating your body and refreshing your mind.

Throughout the day, we all tend to carry a lot of emotional baggage, and breathing exercises can help relieve that stress, and get you in a calm, focused state, which can help you make better decisions. Here is a great video on YouTube about deep breathing: Breathing Relaxation Exercise by David Garrigus.

There are a lot of resources on Yoga available. The library, the internet, books, videos, professional classes, and more that can give you many different and wonderful yoga routines. To get a good idea of a great Yoga routine, check out this video by YogaVidyaEnglish, Yoga for Complete Beginners.

Pet therapy
Pet therapy, as the name suggests, deals with the exposure to pets and animals as a way to lighten your spirits, lift your mood, and get you laughing within no time! A number of studies have found that people who spend more time with their pets are less likely to be affected by depression, anxiety, stress, and even life-threatening cardiovascular disorders. High blood pressure patients, too, have found benefits in pet therapy.

Look at someone who's walking a pet in the garden- you'll find yourself smiling in just seconds- that's the power of pet therapy.

Make it a point to spend some time with your pet-take them out for a walk, feed them or bathe them; play with them or give them treats. If you don't have a pet, then consider getting one!

Hypnotherapy
Hypnotherapy is yet another effective therapy falling under alternative healing practices, and is known to hold amazing benefits for the mind and to aid in better mental function.

While hypnotherapy practices do require the intervention of a professional hypnotherapist, self hypnosis practices allow you to experience the benefits of hypnotherapy at an individual level.

Start a self hypnosis session by lying down in a comfortable position and getting relaxed. Relax every tense muscle in your body and feel your body getting light. Next, allow your mind to focus on an ideal condition- a situation, an event or an occasion that makes you happy (in this case, a situation that would lead to better mood, less stress etc). Focus and hold onto this thought-allow it to come to life in your mind, see yourself laughing and having the best day of your life, and telling yourself this is what you deserve! Let your worries melt away and allow joy, love, and laughter into your life.

Doing this exercise daily for at least a couple of months can make you feel wonderfully at ease- you'll be more energetic, lively, and less prone to stress and anxiety! If you prefer a guided self-hypnosis session, then my favorite place to go is: HypnosisDownloads.

Chapter 4: Laughter Yoga

In the mid 1990's, Dr Madan Kataria, a general physician, realized the importance of laughter and how it could help the body heal and overcome problems, both physical and mental. He then developed a new form of yoga known as laughter yoga, which incorporated techniques of both laughter and yoga, to speed up healing and improve the overall health of an individual.

It all started with a small group of people getting together in a public park and laughing their hearts out. It didn't take long before its popularity spread rapidly. Laughter yoga (now also popularly known as laughter therapy) spread like wildfire and began grabbing the attention of the masses.

One of the best aspects about laughter yoga is the fact that it involves practically no strained movements for the body, and pretty much anyone can do it with ease! Here are some wonderful techniques that can be used to incorporate laughter into your life- and remember, it's all in the mind; even if you fake the laugh, eventually you will get the real benefits from it. So do your body a favor and laugh out loud!

The HaHa HoHo
You want to get in a comfortable sitting position with your legs crossed. Keep your back straight, as straight as you can. Once you're in this position, put your hands over your stomach, placing the palms of your hands on top of each other. Concentrate on your stomach and let out a hearty "Hoho." Afterwards, put your hands over your heart and concentrate on your chest. Then let out a "Haha." Change between the two positions. Start slow and try to speed up to shouts of "Hoho, haha, hoho, haha."

The He Ha Ho Hu
This exercise requires you to be standing. First, put your hands on top of your head and do an inward "Hehehe", to clear your mind of tension. Move your hands from your head to your chest and shout "Hahaha!" Then move your hands onto your stomach and yell "Hohoho!" Finally, focus on your feet and have some fun trampling the ground with your feet and shouting, "Huhuhu."

The Laughing Wave
Think of this exercise as connecting heaven and earth with your laughter. While in a standing position, bow down with your torso and then put your hands palm down towards the ground. Concentrate on the floor. Then, without lifting your torso, twist your arms so that your palms face the sky. While doing this yell out, "Hahahaha."

The Welcome Laughter
This exercise really utilizes the contagious nature of laughter. If in a group, keep eye contact with someone and burst out laughing until everyone is laughing

along. When alone, look into a mirror and welcome yourself with a mirthful laugh.

Stretching Ha's
Simply reach your arms as high as you can. Really stretch so that you can feel the air circulating through your body and laugh "Ha ha ha" for a full minute. You'll be surprised at how good you feel afterwards.

Mantras
Mantras are simply vocal repetitions. Say to yourself, out loud or in your head, something like "Let the world be full of laughter", and imagine the whole world laughing along with you.

Finishing
When it's time to end your yoga laughing exercises, it is time to sit still, preferably cross-legged, connecting the tips of your thumbs with the tips of your fore finger, and sing, "Om." Feel within your body where this sound resonates best. Perform this exercise for at least a minute, or until you feel calm and relaxed.

YouTube is a great source of excellent videos that'll make finding the right exercises for your laughter routine easier-be sure to check them out to get some more laughter into your life.

LAUGHTER YOGA: Intro, Benefits and Exercises by Robert Rivest

Laughter Yoga Steps by Dr. Madan Kataria

Laughter Yoga 40 Foundation Exercises by Robert Rivest

LOOK YOUNGER! w/Happy Face Yoga Facial Exercises by Sigsac

Chapter 5: Mental Strategies For Overcoming Bad Memories

Let's face it- every once in a while, you may get caught up in a situation or an event that's beyond your control- and that's exactly when you need to add some laughter to your life. It is not unusual for people to laugh when they are afraid, uncomfortable, or ashamed. We use laughter as a defense, but also as a way to defuse difficult situations and emotions. It shouldn't be surprising then that many comedians come from difficult childhoods. Below is a quick list of some famous comedians who suffered from traumatic childhoods.

Bill Cosby was raised in the projects with an alcoholic father. This seems kind of amazing considering his creation of The Hit TV show the Huxtables. Chevy Chase lived in constant fear of his abusive mother. Sometimes he was awakened by being repeatedly slapped in the middle of the night. His mother was also known to lock him in the bathroom for hours on end. Richard Pryor was raised in a brothel. His mother was a prostitute and his father was her pimp. Humorist Art Buchwald was raised in seven different foster homes after his mother was committed to a mental institution. He once said, "If you make the bullies laugh, they don't beat you up."

What is it about humor that helps people cope with a difficult past? Does it actually heal us or is it just so enjoyable that it only seems to heal us?

Mental pain is both a psychological and physical process. We know that laughter is good for the body. We already know that there is a negative correlation between laughter and the chances of heart disease, but there are also bio-psychosocial benefits of humor.

When people laugh, parts of their limbic system are activated. Laughter also produces feel good hormones like endorphins. Filling your brain with these endorphins has been seen to lead to surprisingly happy results in all facets of life throughout history.

Psychologists have yet to solidify one theory as to why laughter can help so many people recover from a devastating past. Here are the two main theories:

If a person has had an unhappy childhood, it might help for them to use humor. By accessing painful memories and incorporating them with humor, the patient is in a way, reinventing, or replacing their old memories. In this way laughter creates a new, healthier perspective. With the addition of endorphins that laughter elicits, it makes approaching a difficult past easier.

It might also work in another way. The depression that comes with a traumatic past comes with what is called *learned helplessness*. Researchers found that unusual or constant punishment or neglect, leads to children feeling as if they are unable to change anything, or that if they do try to change their situation, it will only lead to abuse. Being able to laugh at a situation from the past has been shown to be very healing to a variety of different people. The goal is to de-sensitize the painful memory so that you don't keep constantly bringing it up, and if you do, you now remember it as less painful or as a learning experience.

Clinical psychologists have been using this knowledge and developing humor therapies with patients who have suffered from traumatic childhoods. The results have been promising. Below are some things that you can try by yourself.

Writing
Patients with bad childhoods are sometimes asked by their therapist to write about their childhood in a humorous way. This might include making the former perpetrator into a ridiculous monster or creating an extremely idiotic character of someone who might have been around during the time of the abuse but did nothing to help. In this therapy, the patient lets their mind run wild, writing down whatever crazy characteristics or attributes to the painful memory that they feel is necessary to help them feel better. The goal is to do this every time the memory pops up, so that over time, its negative effect is totally destroyed.

Hyperbole
Since approaching a difficult past can be frightening and riddled with anxiety, it sometimes helps if the person minimizes it. This is hyperbole. It is not meant to minimize the actual pain, but rather to make the cause of the pain approachable. The person might say that they are a "just little bit upset" about being abused or they might give their unhappy childhood a name like "less than ideal."

Imagination
Psychologists have found that many patients that have had unhappy childhoods were not allowed to express anger. This manifests itself in an inability to express anger at their past (or even during present situations). Anger, crying, and laughter are three of the most cathartic exercises a person can do. A therapist may ask that a patient pretend that their former perpetrator is a small bug. The patient can then pretend to squash it with their fist then flick it away as if it were nothing but a piece of lint. The scenes can get extremely extravagant, such as imagining a laser gun that zaps the other person or memory to smithereens. You could also imagine yourself in a beautiful garden on a sunny day and burying the painful memory behind a small group of flowers and laughing to yourself while doing it. The key to this is to find something that really makes you smile inside, and then use the imagination to create a scenario that destroys or makes humor of the memory every time that painful memory comes up.

Making a List
Try making a list of insecurities that you know that you need to work on, and then modifying that list for humorous purposes. This allows you to laugh at yourself while minimizing the aspects that you need to work on. For example, if you are insecure about your weight, you could write down: "Wow, I may need to lose

some weight or my family is going to need to rent an elephant just to carry my casket to the grave."

Humor is essential to good health. It boosts the immune system, assists in cardiac function, and relieves tension. Laughter has now been shown to help those struggling with trauma. Psychologists not only use humor to help those overcome an unhappy childhood, but new studies show that laughter helps survival rates in cancer patients and people undergoing organ transplants. Although the reasons for its positive psychological effects is still being speculated on, it has been clear for thousands of years that humor is good for the heart, body, and spirit. Lastly, remember that no situation or condition is permanent- everything is subject to change; remind yourself that when you're dealing with tough situations, make a joke of it, transform the memory in your mind, and learn to laugh and smile about it!

Chapter 6: Encourage Laughter With Nutrition

We all know how our diet plays a major role in shaping our physical and mental health. Nutrition is the key to creating a strong, healthy body, and a perspective that is positive. If you are sick, having trouble sleeping, or suffering from other ailments, people often recommend a change of diet. This is because nutrients are the building blocks of what we actually are and how effectively we can function.

There are foods and teas that help increase the likelihood of finding humor in one's life. No, they don't make you burst out laughing if you take them. What they do is that they lead to a lightened, friendlier mood, and a more relaxed state of mind without making you fall asleep.

One of these nutrients are EFA, or essential fatty acids. EFAs have been linked to lower heart disease and decreased depression and sadness. Foods that are rich in EFAs are usually nuts and seeds like walnuts, hemp, chia, and flaxseeds. There are many ways to consume EFAs. Below are two smoothies that are rich in EFAs.

For both recipes, place all the ingredients below in a blender or food processor for 45 seconds or until smooth.

Orange-Carrot Smoothie
1 ¼ cups carrot juice
1 orange, peeled
3 tbs. ground flaxseed
1 ½ tbs. of raw honey
¼ tsp. of ground allspice (optional)

Blueberry-Chia Smoothie
1 ¼ cup coconut milk beverage
1/3 cup tofu
2 tbs. raw honey or agave
3 tbs. chia seeds
1 cup frozen blueberries.

If this mixture is too thick after two minutes of blending, add more coconut milk or water.

This next one is a recipe for Oatmeal cookies. It's not too surprising that a cookie can add a smile to your life. This one, however, is rich with EFAs.

These cookies take 15 minutes to prepare, about 10 minutes to cook, and makes 2 dozen delicious cookies.

Ingredients:
¾ cup olive oil
1 Tb molasses
1 ½ cup sugar
2 eggs
1 tsp vanilla
1 3/4 cup whole spelt flour
2 cups rolled oats
¼ cup hemp flour
¼ cup flax seed
¼ cup hulled hemp seeds
½ cup dark chocolate chips
1 tsp baking powder
¼ tsp soda

Preheat your oven to 375 degrees. Blend the wet ingredients by mixer or by hand. Then blend the dry ingredients together, and then mix everything together. Put thick spoonfuls of batter onto a cookie sheet that is lined with a light mix of oil and flour. Bake 8 to 10 minutes or until the cookies are just barely browned.

The hemp flour, hemp seeds, and flax seed can be found at any organic food market. These foods are rich in EFAs and can be added to oatmeal for a super healthy meal, along with honey and some fresh berries.

In addition to EFA rich foods and smoothies, there are tea supplements that have been shown to improve mood and increase your chances of finding humor in everyday life. With teas, it is much better to get the loose leafed teas, as they are much richer in taste and sustain their healthy properties longer. With loose leafed teas, you can also mix and match to create your own flavor.

St. John's Wort
St. John's Wort has gotten a lot of publicity lately and with good reason. It has shown in numerous clinical studies to be a natural mood brightener. There are even reports that this herb is as effective at treating moderate depression as some prescription medicines, but with fewer side effects.

Kava-Kava
Kava-Kava (or just Kava) is strong in its anti-anxiety properties. People report having feelings of relaxation, peace, and increased sociability after drinking this tea. Some even report having feelings of euphoria. You have to be careful though, Kava has been known to be habit forming, so it is best used rarely.

Korean Ginseng
Korean Ginseng has simultaneously calming and energizing effects. Chronic drinkers of Korean Ginseng report having lowered stress, improved mood, and increased stamina. It's a great supplement to take during a stressful morning for a happy, vibrant day!

Rhodiola

Rhodialo has been used throughout the years by herbalists to help people defend against stressors. It also decreases fatigue, depression and anxiety, as well as increasing neurotransmitter functions that are crucial to mood regulation.

Chapter 7: All Natural Mood Boosting Foods

Mother Nature seems to have a wonderful way of keeping us happy-no wonder there's so many foods out there that boost our mood in just minutes.

Here are some of the best natural (and not-so-natural) foods that have been scientifically proven to boost mood and ease depression. Pick up any of these at the start of the day (preferably with your breakfast), and you're one step closer to a better mood.

Chocolate

Yes, you read that right! It's a guilty pleasure for many of us, and cocoa beans seem to have a good way of relaxing the nerves and getting us in the 'good' mood. Now, many health-conscious people out there may not be so happy with the idea of grabbing a chocolate whenever they're depressed, but hey, you can always switch to a dark chocolate-it's a good source of essential 'healthy' fats, and is known to improve cardiovascular health too!

And for the record, a small chunk of your favorite chocolate can work as effectively as 3 packs of it- so it's a good idea to go slow and limit your intake on this one.

Mussels

Mussels are a great natural food source with high amounts of vitamin B12, and are known to possess excellent brain-protecting properties. They are also known to contain trace minerals, including iodine, zinc, selenium etc, all of which play a vital role in improving thyroid health, which in turn, keeps your mood balanced.

Bananas

Bananas are a rich source of important nutrients for the body- they are packed with iron, phosphorous, vitamin C, potassium, fiber, vitamin A, vitamin B6, and the important amino acid tryptophan.

The ultimate duo of vitamin B6 and tryptophan is what makes bananas a sure winner- vitamin B6 helps convert tryptophan to serotonin- a hormone that uplifts mood and gets you in the 'happy' zone, and also ensures good sleep. Individuals suffering from insomnia, depression, stress, and anxiety are often advised to consume bananas as a natural approach to handling their condition.

Salmon

Salmon is a good natural source of vitamin D and omega-3 fatty acids, both of which are believed to raise the serotonin levels of the brain, which is responsible for giving you that "feel-good feeling."

What's more, lower levels of vitamin D have been linked to depression, and salmon works by giving you a good dose of this vitamin.

Popcorn

Movie buffs love it, and if you do too, don't shy away- popcorn can actually have some wonderful effects on you! This carbohydrate-rich food can increase your serotonin levels, which in turn can make you feel happier and more relaxed.

Walnuts

Rich in heart-healthy antioxidants, walnuts are an excellent way to kick-start your day with good energy and a mood boost. They contain serotonin boosting magnesium and omega-3 fatty acids which fight anxiety, stress, agitation, insomnia, depression, and other related disorders.

Lentils

A kitchen staple, lentils are complex carbohydrates that help increase the brain's production of serotonin- the feel-good neurotransmitter, just like bananas. What's more, lentils are a good natural source of folate- a deficiency of folate has been linked to an increased risk of depression.

Swiss Chard

Easy to grow in your backyard, this green leafy vegetable is packed with magnesium- an essential nutrient required to boost the body's energy levels and keep depression away. A majority of Americans don't really get their required amount of magnesium- and by simply adding more of this vegetable to your meals, you cannot just prevent a deficiency, but you can also get yourself in a good mood.

Chicken

Yes, you read that right! Chicken, turkey, and other lean meats are excellent natural sources of tryptophan, which encourages the body to produce serotonin, which further promotes good sleep and gives you a good mood boost as well. What's more, both these proteins contain an amino acid called tyrosine, which can reduce the symptoms of depression and improve your mental well-being. Best of all, these meats are very versatile- you can add them to your meals without a second thought!

Spinach

Popeye the sailor man ate this for a reason- spinach doesn't just give your body a needed dose of iron, it does much more. Spinach is believed to be a good source of B vitamins- a deficiency of which has been strongly linked to depression.

Yogurt

A deficiency of vitamin D is linked to a number of health problems, and a bad mood is one of them. A body that lacks in this essential vitamin is thought to be much more prone to irritability, anger, anxiety, fear, and depression. Yogurt can provide your body much needed vitamin D and calcium in its purest form, and can cut down your levels of anxiety and stress.

Oyster

Seafood lovers, it's time to rejoice! Oysters are a good source of essential nutrients including zinc, tyrosine and calcium, all of which are believed to play a role in energy production and mood regulation. Be sure to grab a plate when you're feeling low, and you'll be energetic and at your best in no time!

Chapter 8: I Dare You Not To Smile!

Yes, that's right! To lighten things up, I've put down some crazy and, funny jokes that'll make you smile and cheer you up in no time!

Very Berry
Q: What did one strawberry say to the other strawberry?
A: If you hadn't been so fresh we wouldn't be in this jam!

Farty Beans
Q: Why did the chief only put 239 types of beans in his soup?
A: Because one more would be too farty.

Credit Card
Q: How do you get a herd of elephants to stop charging?
A: Take away their credit cards!

Cover-up
Q: What did the rug say to the floor?
A: Don't move! I got you covered.

Knotted String
A piece of string walks into a bar. When he tries to order, the bartender says, "I don't serve strings here." The string goes outside, ties himself up, and musses his ends. He goes back inside and when he orders the bartenders says "Didn't I just tell you, I don't serve string here?" To which he replies, "I'm a frayed knot."

Bad Luck
Maggie's husband was very sick and slipping in and out of consciousness. Maggie waited on him and kept to his bedside throughout his sickness. One day, when her husband had just regained consciousness, he beckoned for Maggie to come close to him so that he could tell her something.

"Maggie, you have never left me no matter how rough things got. You stood by me when I lost my job, you held my hand when my parents died, and you were at my side even when we lost the house. Even now, when I'm so sick, you are here with me. Do you know what I think?"

Maggie smiled softly. "What's that?"

"I think you're bad luck."

The Ketchup Story
A mother was struggling with a ketchup bottle when the phone rang. She asked her five year old son to answer the phone. She heard her daughter say, "Mommy can't come to the phone now, she's hitting the bottle."

Engagement trouble
When a woman in the office got engaged, one of her colleagues congratulated her and said "the first 10 years are usually the hardest" to which, the woman asked "how long have you been married?" "10 years," she replied.

Anniversary Gift
My wife wanted to go somewhere she's never been before for our anniversary, so I brought her to the kitchen.

Politician Trouble
Diapers and politicians have two things in common. They need to be changed regularly and for the same reason.

Good Evening
The evening news is where they begin each segment with "Good evening" then go on to tell you why it isn't.

Beautiful You
A couple went for a dinner at an expensive restaurant. Midway between the meal, the husband complimented the wife and said "you look beautiful tonight." The wife went all blushy and red, when suddenly the husband said "we must get these lights."

Bill Issues
My doctor told me I have six months to live. I told him I couldn't pay the bill, so he gave me six more.

Surprise!
Biology Teacher- In this box, I have a 10 foot long snake.
Student- Snakes don't have feet teacher, you told us that just yesterday!

Madly in Love!
When do you know a guy's in love? When you see him losing interest in his car after a couple of days.

Job Trouble
My job is safe and secure- no one else wants it!

God Wonders
Why did God create Adam before Eve? Because he didn't need instructions on how to create Adam.

A child's play
The parents of a 6-year old boy rushed to the school when they were informed that their child had a terrible cough and was vomiting. The school doctor performed an exam and asked the kid "what's bothering you the most?" to which, the child replied "I must, say-my little sister."

Conclusion

Well now you know. You know the outrageously healthy effects laughter can have on the body, the brain, and on the heart. It is an overall spirit lifter and is an important addition to a healthier, happier life.

You also now know how to increase the amount of laughter in your life. Remember to enjoy your imagination and let it run free every now and then, especially to battle the memories and traumas not wanted from the past. Also, remember that laughing is contagious, and to give it, you also need to share it, and thereby help others to live a healthier and happier life.

Be sure to remember that a healthy diet with the correct foods in it can keep you in the right mood to allow humor and laughter to easily come through in your life, especially if you are trying. You also have learned the incredible benefits of laughter yoga, so be sure to do this as often as possible. Feel free to use your laughter as a mighty shield of joy in your travels through life. So laugh it up baby, you've got no reason not to!

I hope this book was able to help you to find a more fulfilling and happier lifestyle by using the power of laughter.

Finally, if you discovered at least one thing that has helped you or that you think would be beneficial to someone else, be sure to take a few seconds to easily post a quick positive review. As an author, your positive feedback is desperately needed. Your highly valuable five star reviews are like a river of golden joy flowing through a sunny forest of mighty trees and beautiful flowers! *To do your good deed in making the world a better place by helping others with your valuable insight, just leave a nice review.*

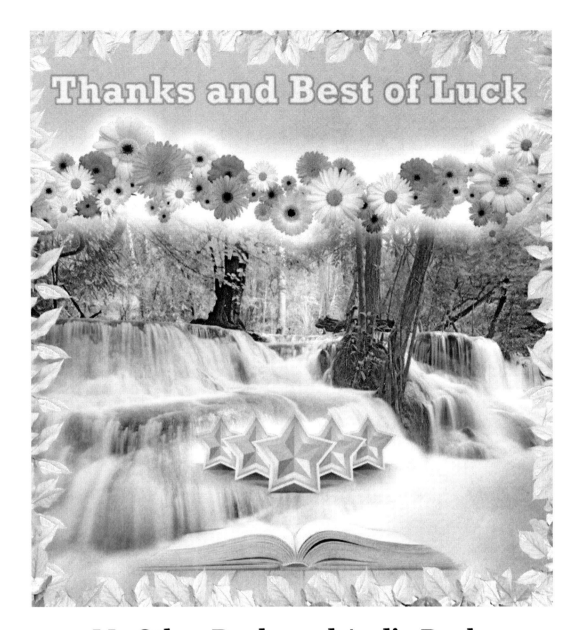

My Other Books and Audio Books
www.AcesEbooks.com

Health Books

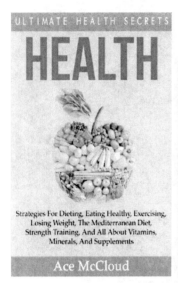

ULTIMATE HEALTH SECRETS

HEALTH

Strategies For Dieting, Eating Healthy, Exercising, Losing Weight, The Mediterranean Diet, Strength Training, And All About Vitamins, Minerals, And Supplements

Ace McCloud

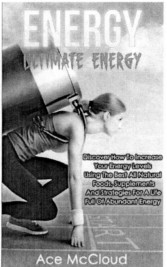

ENERGY
ULTIMATE ENERGY

Discover How To Increase Your Energy Levels Using The Best All Natural Foods, Supplements And Strategies For A Life Full Of Abundant Energy

Ace McCloud

RECIPE BOOK

The Best Food Recipes That Are Delicious, Healthy, Great For Energy And Easy To Make

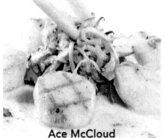

Ace McCloud

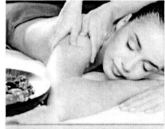

MASSAGE THERAPY

TRIGGER POINT THERAPY
ACUPRESSURE THERAPY
Learn The Best Techniques For Optimum Pain Relief And Relaxation

Ace McCloud

LOSE WEIGHT

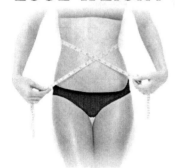

THE TOP 100 BEST WAYS TO LOSE WEIGHT QUICKLY AND HEALTHILY

Ace McCloud

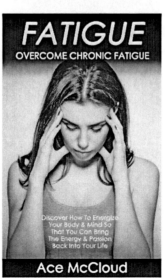

FATIGUE
OVERCOME CHRONIC FATIGUE

Discover How To Energize Your Body & Mind So That You Can Bring The Energy & Passion Back Into Your Life

Ace McCloud

Peak Performance Books

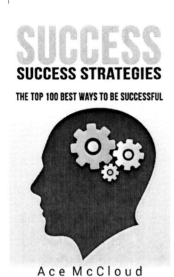

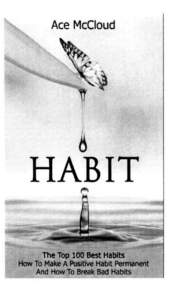

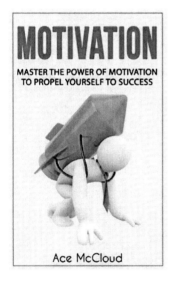

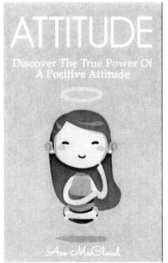

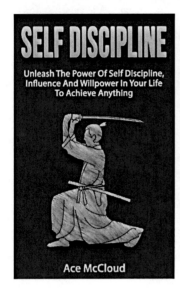

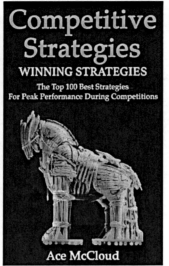

Be sure to check out my audio books as well!

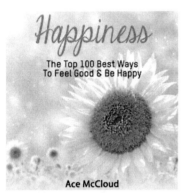

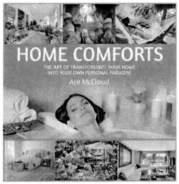

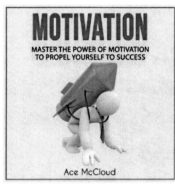

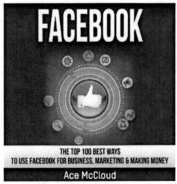

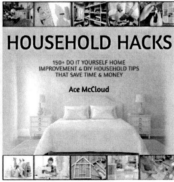

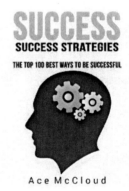

Check out my website at: www.AcesEbooks.com for a complete list of all of my books and high quality audio books. I enjoy bringing you the best knowledge in the world and wish you the best in using this information to make your journey through life better and more enjoyable! **Best of luck to you!**

CPSIA information can be obtained
at www.ICGtesting.com
Printed in the USA
LVOW09s1311220917
549726LV00004B/160/P